10 MINUTES
FACE YOGA EXERCISE

Life-Changing facial Exercises for Younger, Smoother Skin

Sharon C. Schwab

INTRODUCTION

In the fast-paced, stressful world that we live in today, it can be hard to take care of your skin. Stress and pollution wreak havoc on our faces, making us look older than what we are. Yoga is a great way to decompress and relieve stress from everyday life - but did you know that there are specific yoga exercises for your face? In this blog post, I'm going to teach you 5 minutes life-changing face yoga exercises for younger, smoother skin. This is a book we were all waiting for! I hope you enjoy it and find something that works for your lifestyle. A few of the benefits are: better sleep, increased energy, and lower stress levels - what more could you ask for? The first exercise is called "The warmup." It's perfect because it can be done anywhere with no special equipment required. You'll need to do this one in the morning as well as evening time (after work) before bedtime so your body gets used to being on this natural schedule! Let's get started!

CHAPTER ONE

PART 1

What is face yoga exercise?

The term face yoga is a combination of the word "face" and the original practice that was developed in India, Yoga. The concept behind this movement is to train your facial muscles with gentle moves such as smiling or puckering up for an extended period of time while simultaneously stretching them out. These exercises can be done anywhere at any time so you can fit them into your daily routine easily. There are many different types of smiles which work on various areas around the mouth, eyes, forehead and nose but all have one thing in common they will make you feel relaxed!

Effects of Face yoga on you.

Face yoga exercise has been known to help rejuvenate skin by increasing circulation just below its surface because when we smile our cheeks become flushed with blood. This increase in blood flow naturally brings more nutrients and oxygen, which help to brighten our complexion. Not only that but it also stimulates the muscles beneath your skin's top layer (the subcutaneous fat) so you can expect facial contours to become fuller with regular practice of face yoga exercise!

Who should do this?

Face Yoga is suitable for everyone at any age because we all have muscles around our eyes, mouth and forehead! The best part about these exercises is that they require no equipment or special skills just a smile ready to be utilized whenever necessary. These movements might seem simple but don't underestimate their benefits; not only will you look refreshed if done regularly but you'll feel happier too.

How to do the exercises

Pinch your nose, then pull it to the left and hold for 30 seconds. Repeat on other side.

This exercise is great because you can do it anywhere at any time! If you're walking down a street or sitting in the car as a passenger with your seatbelt on during rush hour traffic, just give this easy stretch an attempt! You'll be amazed by how quickly it tones up those facial muscles and tightens tired skin around your eyes giving you that healthy glow we all want so badly.

Face Yoga Poses: Pinched Nose Pose (Nasikagra Mudra) & Eye Mask Stretch (Neti Jihva Bandha Sarvanga).

The pinched nose pose opens up your sinuses and improves blood circulation, which helps reduce dark circles under your eyes. And don't worry about the odd looks you might get, nobody is watching!

The eye mask stretch gives a beautiful lift to tired skin around the eyes by draining away all of that pooled fluid in those delicate tissues - reducing puffiness and fine lines at the same time!

Try this face yoga technique every morning for one week and see how it changes not only your appearance but also how awake you feel throughout the day. This simple exercise will make sure that you never look overworked again!

Facial exercises are often overlooked as an important part of our beauty regimen because most people think they're too difficult or simply unnecessary to do on a daily basis. However, just like your regular workouts at the gym, face yoga can give you a beautiful youthful appearance as well as that amazing self-confidence that comes from always looking our best!

The pinched nose pose is great for draining away all of those fluids which cause dark circles under the eyes and fine lines around them. Just imagine how much better we will look when we're able to cut out all of these age-related issues from our lives so easily? And because it's such an easy technique to do anywhere with anyone watching (we won't tell if you don't!), there really aren't any excuses not to try this exercise on a daily basis!

How Often: Try three times every day - once in the morning, once in the afternoon and then again at night before you go to bed.

Face yoga is not a complicated series of exercises that require hours out of your day - many can be done while sitting in front of the TV or listening to music! It's really up to you how much time you're willing to invest into getting beautiful skin as well as better overall health. We know we'll always make sure that our daily face yoga routine gets completed because it's just so easy when most techniques only take about ten minutes max!

My Experience with Facial yoga exercise

I've never been one for extensive beauty regimens which involve spending an hour doing all sorts of impossible stretches followed by another few hours rubbing expensive creams into my face every single morning... So when I heard about face yoga from a friend of mine, I was really unsure if this would be the simple exercise routine that I've been looking for.

Face yoga is amazing because it only takes ten minutes out of your day to complete (not including any time spent in front of the mirror practicing) - and doesn't require you doing anything too strenuous or physically demanding! You can easily do these exercises while walking down a street, sitting on public transport or even lying in bed before falling asleep at night. That's why we think everyone should give face yoga a try - what have you got to lose?

Face Yoga Exercises are great way to get younger skin with less expensive creams potions without spending hours every day applying them.

Risks and precautions of this practice?

There are no serious risks or precautions associated with face yoga. Some people might find it uncomfortable to do the poses, especially in the beginning. In addition, if you have sensitive skin and/or allergies, some of these exercises might not be a good idea for your particular condition as that can cause additional problems such as redness from rubbing too hard on the cheeks. You should also avoid any exercises that involve lying flat on your back; this is considered dangerous during pregnancy. Lastly, never use heavyweights around your head when doing facial exercises because there's always a risk of injury due to falling over while exercising without proper balance – so don't go overboard!

Why you should try it for yourself!

There are a lot of reasons to give face yoga exercises a try. For one, it feels amazing! The pressure and the stretching can be quite relaxing for most people. It also increases blood flow as well as lymphatic drainage, which both help support healthier-looking skin when performed regularly over time. If you're an actor or model working on your facial expressions then practicing these moves will definitely benefit your career by keeping those muscles toned and strong. And let's not forget about anti-aging benefits like reduced wrinkles and fine lines around the eyes, mouth & forehead area (where signs of aging typically show up first).

Possible side effects? When done improperly without maintaining proper technique or engaging in suitable breathing techniques during practice certain possible side effects can include muscle soreness, nose bleeds, and/or a headache. If you are experiencing any of these side effects stop practicing immediately & consult your doctor or face

yoga instructor before trying again!

CHAPTER TWO

PART 2

The warmup

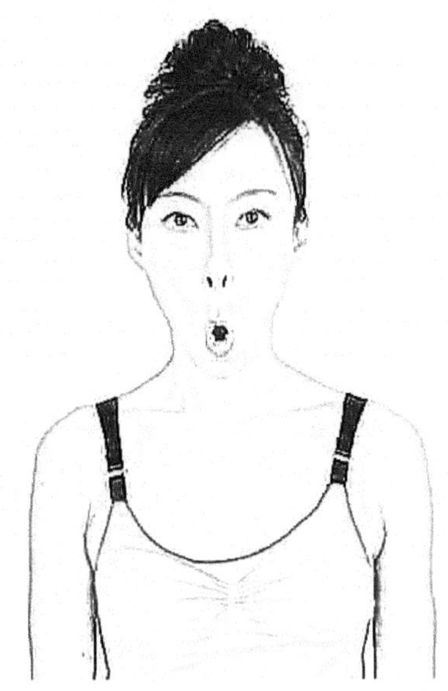

STEPS:

This is a great position for all-over blood circulation.

Drop your jaw as though yawning, and feel the sensation in your cheeks.

Move your gaze from eye-level to the ceiling without moving your forehead muscles.

Hold for 10 seconds, breathing throughout.

Repeat twice for 30 seconds.

For the neck.

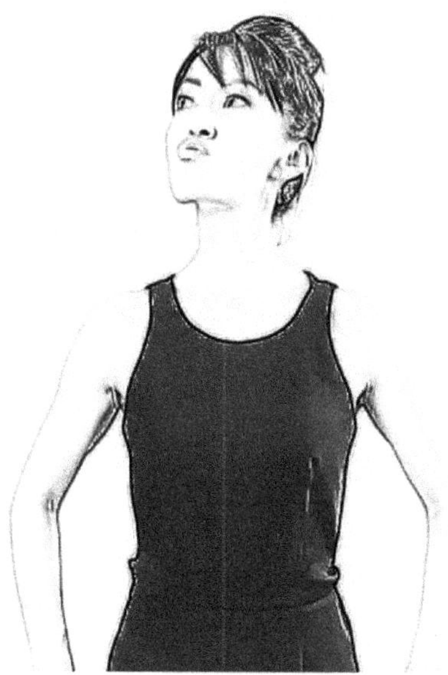

STEPS:

This position relieves stress and tones the neck. Because the platysma muscle connects the neck and mouth, this stretch can help tone your jawline. Move your chin to one side, slightly up at a 45-degree angle, while relaxing your shoulders. Make a kiss by puckering your lips.

Hold for 10 seconds while remembering to breathe.

Repeat on the other side.

Repeat on both sides for a total of 30 seconds on each side.

For the forehead.

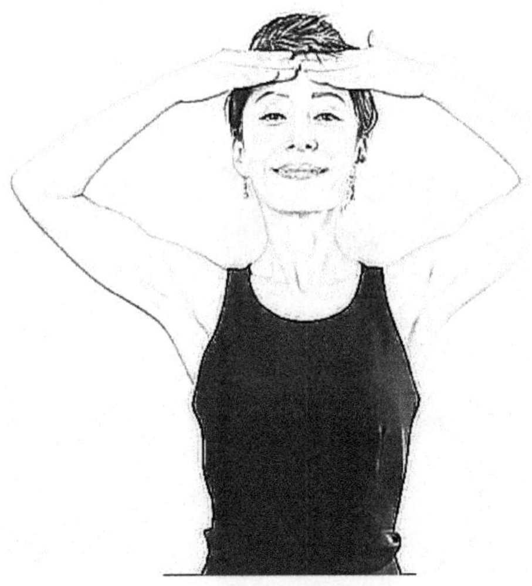

This is known as the "quick pick-me-up" position. That's because it also serves as a meditation, as you accept the energy of your surroundings (great for a morning face yoga ritual).

Make a downward V-shape with your fingers on your brow, pushing up slightly. Breathe in and out for 10 seconds,

Breathe in and out for 10 seconds,

Close your eyes and enjoy the sensation as you run your palms along the sides of your face.

Repeat this process two more times for a total of 30 seconds.

For the eyes.

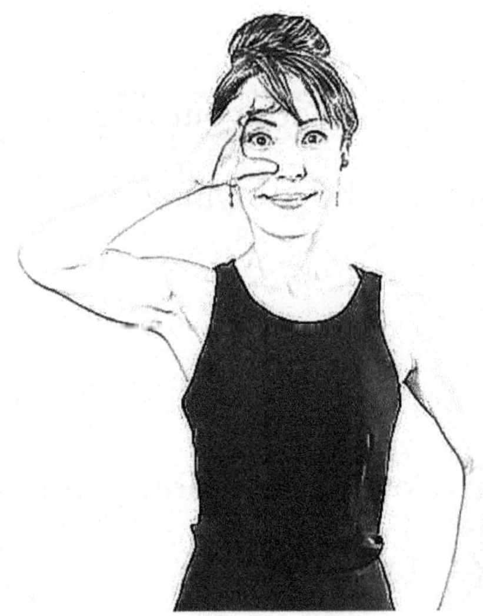

This position separates the lower lid movement as well as the forehead muscles to target the sensitive under-eye region. Try not to furrow your brow.

Form a "C" with your hand. Position your index fingers over the brow and along the upper eye bones.

Place your thumb directly above the nostril on the side of your nose. Make a downward and then a sideways motion with your fingers.

Open your eyes as wide as you can while keeping your shoulders relaxed. Hold for five seconds while pressing your index finger firmly into your brow and keeping your brow and forehead still.

Close your eyes and relax for a few seconds after squinting five times.

Repeat this process two more times for a total of 30 seconds. Rep on the other side.

For the mouth.

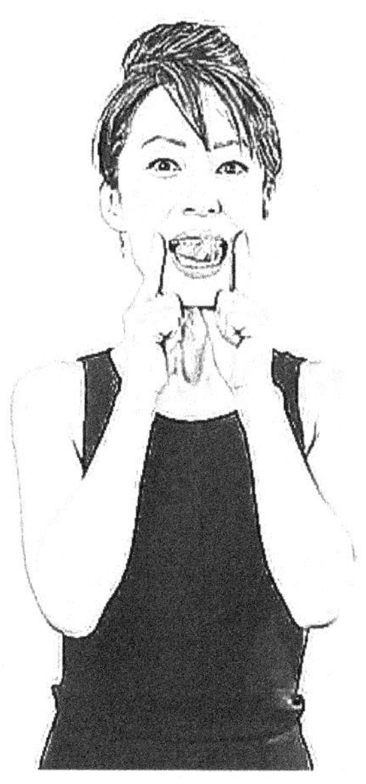

STEPS:

Lips, as we all know, thin as we age owing to collagen loss. This position stimulates the lip barrier, resulting in naturally full, luscious lips.

Put your index fingers on the sides of your lips.

Show off your complete row of front teeth by smiling.

Check that the corners of your mouth are all at the same level.

Curl your tongue slightly and slowly shift it to one side for 5 seconds. Move your tongue to the opposite side for 5 seconds.

Repeat twice more for a total of 30 seconds, remembering to breathe at all times.

CHAPTER THREE

PART 3

The Brow-Raiser

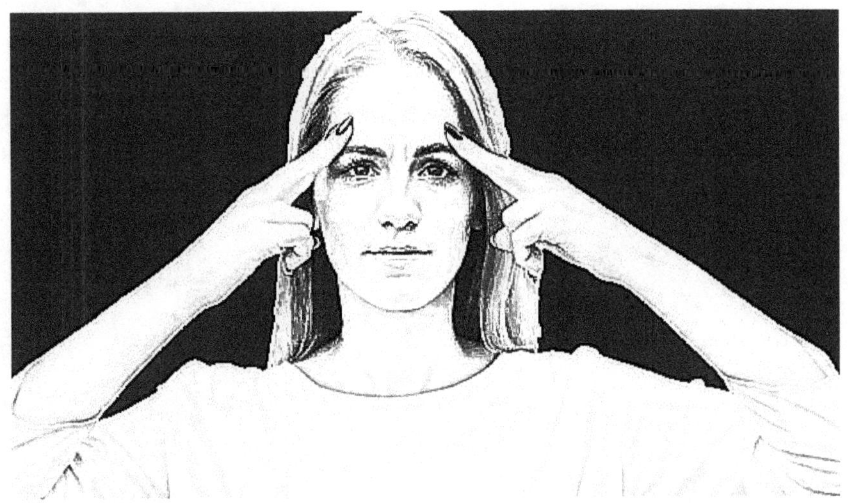

Use this face workout on a daily basis to keep your brows up where they belong:

STEPS:

1. Make a closed peace sign with your index and middle fingers.

2. Place your fingernails between your brows and gently press the skin down.

3. Raise and lower your brows, generating resistance with the weight of your fingernails.

4. Repeat 10 times more.

5. Finish all six sets

Tip: Include IRIS in your face exercise to address aging symptoms around the eye contour.

The Cheekbone Lift

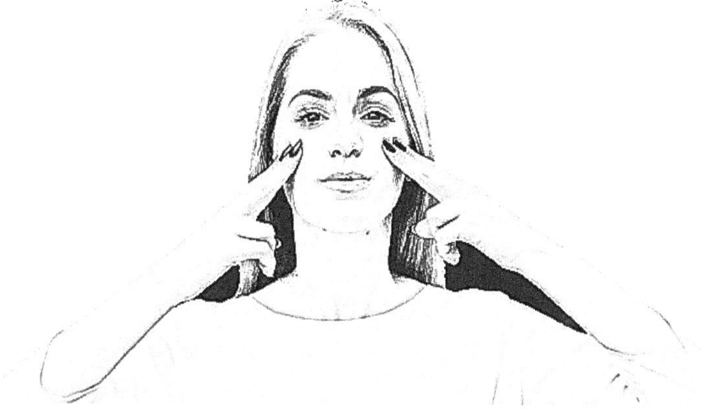

We weren't all born with Angelina-Jolie-as-Maleficent cheekbones, but face exercises might help you come closer. Follow these techniques to swap out flabby, chubby cheeks for sculpted cheekbones:

STEPS:

1. Run your fingertips down each cheekbone.

2. Gently pull the skin taut.

3. Form an extended "O" with your lips; you should feel resistance in your cheek muscles.

4. Maintain for 5 seconds

5. Finish 10-15 sets

The Chipmunk Cheek Squeeze

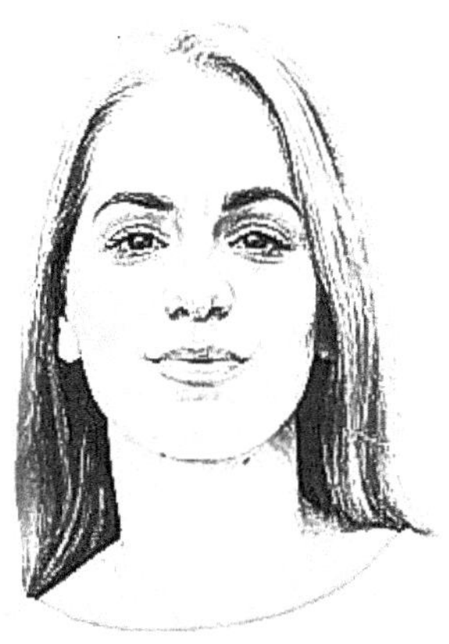

Sculpting big cheeks and an excuse to make the same fish expression over and again? Please sign us up. Here's how to get rid of those acorn-storage pouches:

STEPS:

1. Tilt your head back and press your chin forward.

2. Suck in your cheeks as much as you can.

3. Maintain for 5 seconds

4. Finish 10-15 sets

The Jaw Flex

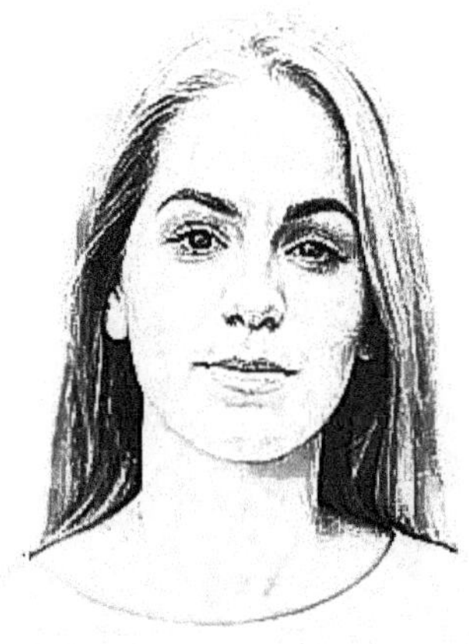

A double chin might make you appear larger and older than you are. With this face workout, you may reduce facial fat and get a more defined appearance:

STEPS:

1. Tilt your head back and stare at the ceiling.

2. Cross your lower lip as far as you can across your top lip; you should feel this in the jaw muscles around your ears.

3. Maintain for 10 seconds

4. Finish 10-15 sets

The Puffer Fish Press

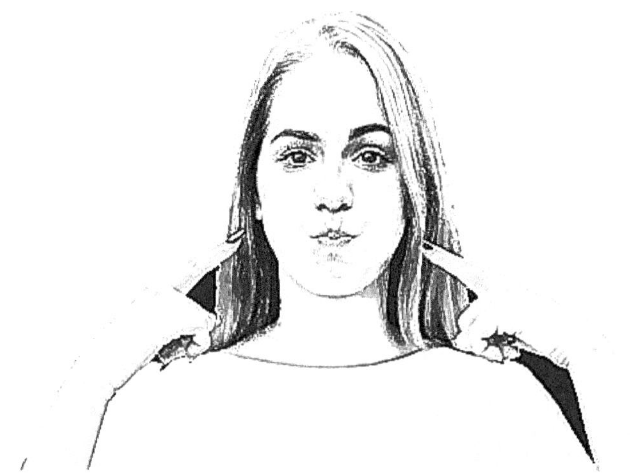

This face workout can help you get rid of those unfunny laugh lines around your lips. As an example, consider the following:

STEPS:

1. Squeeze your cheeks and close your lips.

2. Move the air from one cheek to the other.

3. Move the air from one cheek to the other for 30 seconds.

Use the anti-aging side of your LUNA to massage away any tension after your face workouts, just like you would with a foam roller after a typical workout.

CHAPTER FOUR

PART 4

Air Blowing

Try this easy Yoga for a Beautiful Face to decrease chubbiness on your face.

What to Do:

Inhale as much air into your mouth as you can.

Shift the air in your mouth from one side of your cheek to the other, as if you were cleaning your teeth with mouthwash.

Benefits:

Best Yoga for Burning Fat on the Face

Your face will be contoured as a result of this.

Reduces puffiness in the cheeks

Puckering of the Lips

The goal of this face yoga approach is to tone your chin muscles and minimize your double chin.

What to Do:

Bring your lower lip across your top lip, bringing it as near to your nose as possible.

Hold this position for at least 15 seconds.

Repeat this process ten times.

While performing this workout, one may experience little jaw discomfort.

Benefits:

Reduces the appearance of a double chin

Enhances the suppleness of the skin around your mouth

Sculpts your jaw line

Protruding Cheeks

Another workout that may be done to define your face is Sunken Cheeks. This can be done even while drinking through a straw. This is the greatest Yoga for reducing wrinkles on the face.

What to Do:

Suck in your cheeks so that the muscles on both sides sink in.

Remain in this posture for 15 seconds and then repeat at least ten times.

Benefits:

It raises your jaw line.

Increases the chubbiness of your face

Make your face appear younger.

Exercises for the Nasolabial Fold

Here's an activity to help with the lines around your mouth.

What Should I Do?

With your mouth open, take in as much air as you can.

Pull your cheeks in as much as you can while doing so.

Then, slowly expel the air from your mouth.

Benefits:

Reduces the appearance of wrinkles around the mouth

Sculpts your jaw line

Ensures that the laugh lines are under control.

Observation of Objects

This is an excellent eye yoga pose.

What to Do:

Keep your eyes open and your brows raised to reduce wrinkles.

Hold this position for a few seconds.

Concentrate your attention on a point in front of you.

Repeat this process at least 5 times.

Benefits:

Removes crow's feet

Skin around the eyes is toned.

Enhances the elasticity of the skin around the eyes

Broad grin

This is yet another face skin tightening yoga that targets the cheek muscles.

What to Do:

Smile as wide as you can, revealing all of your teeth.

Hold this posture for a few seconds before repeating 15-20 times.

Benefits:

Best Yoga for a Slimmer Face

This product tightens the skin around your mouth.

Stretches the skin on the back of your neck

Enhances elasticity

Eyes Closed

If you have fine lines and wrinkles around your eyes, try this anti-aging face yoga to tone and tighten them up.

What Should I Do?

Pull your index finger upwards, keeping it on the outer corners of your eyes, so that your cheeks are pushed up in a grin.

Hold this for a few seconds before relaxing.

The workout below focuses on eliminating wrinkles and giving the face a more youthful appearance.

Benefits:

Effortlessly removes wrinkles around the eyes

Removes tiny wrinkles and crow's feet

Facial Stretching

A fantastic yoga for a younger-looking face that may relax facial muscles and enhance skin elasticity:

What Should I Do?

Maintain your index fingers on either side of your eyes and your thumbs on either side of your lips.

Pull your skin up with your fingertips.

You'd sense a strain in your muscles.

Hold it for a few seconds, then relax and repeat.

Benefits:

It provides an immediate facial lift.

Skin is tightened as a result of using this product.

Tone your jawline and cheek lines

Scrunch Your Face

This is an excellent yoga for a clear face, as well as for relaxing your muscles and toning your skin.

What Should I Do?

Maintain a comfortable sitting position and breathe deeply.

Make a fist with your palms.

Close your eyelids as firmly as possible, scrunching the facial muscles.

Benefits:

Reduces stress-related symptoms

Enhances blood circulation

Internal tension is relieved.

Stick your tongue out

Following on from the last exercise, here's how to decrease facial fat using Yoga:

What Should I Do?

Exhale through your mouth and extend your tongue.

Keep your palms and eyes open.

Repeat the process 3-4 times more.

Benefits:

Burns fat on the cheeks

It stretches the muscles in your jaw.

Reduces the appearance of a double chin

Face of a Balloon

Another yoga facelift practice that might help with chubbiness and toning the region around your mouth.

What Should I Do?

Keep your mouth closed and your lips pushed together.

Blow air into the area behind your top lip and hold it for 10 counts.

Shift the air to your left cheek for 10 seconds and hold it there.

Do the same thing with your right cheek. This exercise should be repeated at least 10-15 times.

Benefits:

Stretches all of your face's regions equally

Reduces facial puffiness

Tightens the muscles in your mouth and jaws.

The Fish Face Experiment

This is a simple workout that will transform your face into that of a fish.

What Should I Do?

Suck your cheeks in, make a fish face with your lips, and try to grin.

Remain in this posture for a few seconds before repeating 5 times.

Benefits:

Stretches the region around your neck and chin

Contours your face and gives it a sculpted appearance

Chin Raised

Do you want a defined jaw line and toned cheeks? Here's one of the most effective face yoga exercises for a double chin.

What Should I Do?

Raise your face to the ceiling and blow air out of your mouth.

Repeat this process for a few seconds.

Benefits:

Tones the neck region

Reduces the appearance of a double chin

Increases stiffness in the cheek and jaw areas

Tongue-in-Chief

This yoga for face tightening practice may cause some discomfort in your jaw, but it is really useful for strengthening your facial muscles.

What Should I Do?

Experiment with sticking your tongue out.

Make an attempt to contact your chin with your tongue.

Hold this posture for a total of 10 seconds.

Return to your original location.

Benefits:

Muscle tension is relieved.

It helps to strengthen the jawline.

Tone the skin around your eyes and mouth.

Stretch Your Legs

Do this easy workout to strengthen all of your face muscles.

What Should I Do?

Keep your index and middle fingers on both cheekbones.

Pull your skin up to your eyes now.

Now expand your mouth to make an oval shape.

Hold for a few seconds, then relax and try again.

Benefits:

All of your face muscles are stretched.

Enhances the suppleness of your skin

Raises your brows

You might try chewing gum in addition to these face yoga exercises. This is an excellent technique to shape and define your jawline. To see results, you must perform these workouts on a regular basis. It is also critical to maintain a healthy lifestyle and nutrition. Consume a lunch of fresh fruits and vegetables, as well as lots of water. If you follow these recommendations faithfully, you will gradually but steadily be able to reverse the effects of the aging process!

CONCLUSION

Face Yoga is a physical and mental exercise that can improve your mood, reduce anxiety, help with weight loss, or just make you feel more relaxed. In this book, we've provided the basics of what face yoga is all about as well as some side effects of doing it incorrectly. We hope to have helped clear up any confusion by providing some common questions people may have when considering whether they would like to try this for themselves!

With all of the benefits and side effects, you may be wondering why anyone would want to try this. Well, we recommend trying face yoga exercises for yourself because it's an easy way to reduce wrinkles! Whether your goal is reducing wrinkles or just feeling more energized throughout your day, taking some time out each week to do these simple facial movements will help you achieve that. Join us in our quest to live a better life by living healthier lives with regular exercise!

And it also improves blood circulation which is helpful for the skin! You don't need any fancy equipment or expensive treatments because this type of exercise has been around since the time of ancient Chinese medicine. So why not give it a try?